Rebeca Bastos Vasconcelos Marinho
Clarissa Pessoa Fernandes Forte

Hypertension and the dental treatment of hypertensive patients

Rebeca Bastos Vasconcelos Marinho
Clarissa Pessoa Fernandes Forte

Hypertension and the dental treatment of hypertensive patients

Dentistry for Patients with Special Needs

ScienciaScripts

Imprint
Any brand names and product names mentioned in this book are subject to trademark, brand or patent protection and are trademarks or registered trademarks of their respective holders. The use of brand names, product names, common names, trade names, product descriptions etc. even without a particular marking in this work is in no way to be construed to mean that such names may be regarded as unrestricted in respect of trademark and brand protection legislation and could thus be used by anyone.

Cover image: www.ingimage.com

This book is a translation from the original published under ISBN 978-613-9-61628-2.

Publisher:
Sciencia Scripts
is a trademark of
Dodo Books Indian Ocean Ltd. and OmniScriptum S.R.L publishing group

120 High Road, East Finchley, London, N2 9ED, United Kingdom
Str. Armeneasca 28/1, office 1, Chisinau MD-2012, Republic of Moldova, Europe
Printed at: see last page
ISBN: 978-620-7-88056-0

Table of contents:

REBECA BASTOS VASCONCELOS MARINHO

HYPERTENSION AND DENTAL TREATMENT OF HYPERTENSIVE PATIENTS

FORTALEZA

2018

SUMMARY

Systemic arterial hypertension is a cardiovascular disease characterized by abnormally high blood pressure equal to or greater than 140/90 mmHg, which affects a large part of the world's population. There are various causes for its onset, which can be primary or secondary. This condition is considered to be one of the most important risk factors for the development of various cardiovascular and cerebrovascular diseases and for kidney failure. With the increase in life expectancy and advances in medicine around the world, the number of elderly patients with systemic diseases such as hypertension is becoming more and more frequent in the dental office, making it essential for dental surgeons to have knowledge of clinical medicine to enable them to manage this type of patient properly and safely. The aim of this study is to review the literature on hypertension and the care that should be taken during the dental treatment of hypertensive patients seen by general dental surgeons. The patient's stage of hypertension should be taken into account, as well as checking the medications administered and other associated comorbidities through a thorough anamnesis. Anxiety is also a factor that can predispose to a rise in blood pressure, which can be well managed through iatrosedation or pharmacosedation. If it is not possible to achieve acceptable blood pressure levels, the patient should be rescheduled. Blood pressure changes during dental treatment can vary according to the patient's fear when undergoing the dental procedure, especially in the moments before the administration of the local anesthetic solution, whether with or without vasoconstrictor, which should not exceed the use of two tubes. When considering patients who use antihypertensive drugs, the possible oral complications caused by them, such as hyposalivation, xerostomia and especially gingival hyperplasia, should be noted. Knowledge of antihypertensive drugs is important so that dentists are aware of possible drug interactions in order to avoid them. From the diagnosis to the treatment of hypertension, the dental surgeon must know how to identify the factors that lead to a hypertensive crisis and be able to conduct the treatment with a view to avoiding them through changes in dental treatment, such as scheduling appointments in the morning, selecting anesthetics and the appropriate amount for the case. It is also important, in the event of a crisis, to know how to differentiate between urgency and emergency, bearing in mind the best course of action to take in the event of a crisis. In short, in order to be able to intervene clinically safely and effectively in these patients, the general dental surgeon must be aware of the patient's medical condition and how to modify the dental treatment.

Keywords: Systemic arterial hypertension. Ambulatory blood pressure monitoring. Dentistry.

Chapter 1

1 INTRODUCTION

Systemic arterial hypertension (SAH) is a multifactorial clinical condition characterized by high and sustained levels of blood pressure (BP). It is often associated with alterations in the functional and/or structural clinical conditions of the target organs (heart, brain, kidneys and blood vessels) and metabolic alterations, with a consequent increase in the risk of fatal and non-fatal cardiovascular events (Sociedade Brasileira de Cardiologia, 2006; WILLIAMS, 2010). Its pathogenesis is complex and includes a high incidence of obesity, salt sensitivity and activation of the renin-angiotensin-aldosterone system. This complexity requires a therapeutic combination that includes changes in eating habits and appropriate antihypertensive regimens (ORTEGA; SEDKI; ENAYER, 2015).

SAH is diagnosed by detecting high and sustained levels of BP through its casual or programmed measurement to confirm the diagnosis. The measurement of blood pressure (BP) should be carried out in every evaluation by doctors of any specialty and other health professionals, whether in the public or private sphere.

Mortality from cardiovascular disease (CVD) increases progressively as BP rises above 115/75mmHg in a linear, continuous and independent manner (BRAZILIAN CARDIOLOGICAL SOCIETY, 2009). It is considered one of the main modifiable risk factors for cardiovascular disease, kidney disease and stroke, and one of the most important public health problems. In Brazil, it affects more than 30 million Brazilians, half of whom are unaware that they are ill (SOCIEDADE BRASILEIRA DE HIPERTENSÂO, 2010).

According to the World Report on Non-Communicable Diseases (WHO) in 2010, the main causes of death from non-communicable diseases in 2008 were: cardiovascular diseases (17 million deaths, or 48%); cancer (7.6 million, or 21%); and respiratory diseases, including asthma and chronic obstructive pulmonary disease (COPD), (4.2 million). In 2009, Global health risks (WHO) reported that, worldwide, high blood pressure is the estimated cause of 7.5 million deaths, around 12.8% of all annual deaths. In 2001, around 7.6 million deaths in the world were attributed to high blood pressure (54% from strokes and 47% from ischemic heart disease), with the majority being individuals from low and medium economic development and more than half being between 45 and 69 years old (WILLIAMS, 2010). However, the influence of socioeconomic status on the occurrence of SAH is complex and difficult to establish (CONEN, *et al.,* 2009). In Brazil, SAH is more prevalent among individuals with less schooling and CVD has been identified as the leading cause of death worldwide. In 2007, there were 308,466 deaths from diseases of the circulatory system (MALTA *et al.*, 2009). CVDs are also responsible for a high frequency of hospitalizations, causing high medical and socio-economic costs (Sociedade Brasileira de Cardiologia, 2009).

The 1995 Public Health Notebook reported that the prevalence of hypertension increased progressively with age and that it was related to skin color, family history of hypertension and behavioral habits, as well as verifying that hypertensive women controlled their BP levels better than hypertensive men in all age groups (KLEIN et al., 1995). A study published in 2008 confirms that there is a direct and linear relationship between BP and age, with the prevalence of hypertension in the over-65 age group being over 60% (CESARINO *et al*, 2008). The Brazilian Society of Cardiology also adds that cardiovascular risk factors often come together: genetic predisposition and environmental factors tend to contribute to this combination in families with an unhealthy lifestyle.

According to the World Health Organization (2003), in order to control and prevent chronic conditions, people need to be informed about them, motivated to change long-term behaviors and prepared to self-manage their chronic condition. From this perspective, the intervention of health professionals such as dental surgeons has been aimed at achieving the population's adherence to health promotion and recovery care, as well as primary and secondary prevention in the face of actual or potential illness.

Dental surgeons often provide dental care to hypertensive patients, as this is a cardiovascular disease with a high prevalence (22% to 41% of the Brazilian population) (IV BRAZILIAN GUIDELINES ON ARTERIAL HYPERTENSION), and this professional needs to take into account the influence that treatment will have on the patient's blood pressure. It is necessary to consider the precautions related to the use of local anesthetic solutions, as well as the importance of anxiety control, pain control, knowledge of emergency maneuvers to remove patients from hypertensive crisis, knowledge of medications in use and the adverse effects of these medications, which can cause oral and/or systemic alterations. Drug interactions should also be taken into account, as their incorrect use can aggravate the patient's hypertension (OLIVEIRA, SIMONE, RIBEIRO, 2010). Thus, knowledge of the patient's general health conditions through a well-conducted anamnesis, physical examination and contact with the doctor responsible for the patient, when necessary, are fundamental for a correct diagnosis and appropriate therapy (SHCAIRA, 2005).

In this context, dental surgeons must be aware that they may have patients in their work environment with diagnosed or undiagnosed hypertension who could potentially develop medical emergencies, such as a hypertensive crisis. It is therefore necessary for the dental surgeon to be intellectually and technically prepared to treat these patients and avoid any emergency event that may occur before, during or after dental care. Based on the above, the aim of this study is to carry out a literature review on systemic arterial hypertension and the dental treatment of patients with this disease, aimed at general dental surgeons.

Chapter 2

2 PREPOSITION

2.1 General Objective

To review the literature on hypertension and the care that should be taken during the dental treatment of hypertensive patients seen by general dental surgeons.

2.2 Specific objectives

- To review the literature on hypertension, looking for current national and international data on the epidemiology, classification, etiology, associated comorbidities and medical treatment of this disease.
- To provide up-to-date information that can help the general practitioner in the planning and dental treatment of hypertensive patients.

Chapter 3

3 LITERATURE REVIEW

3.1 General description

Arterial hypertension is a multifactorial disease conceptualized as a syndrome, characterized by the presence of high blood pressure levels associated with metabolic and hormonal alterations and trophic phenomena (cardiac and vascular hypertrophy) (BRAZILIAN HYPERTENSION SOCIETY; BRAZILIAN CARDIOLOGY SOCIETY; BRAZILIAN NEPHROLOGY SOCIETY, 2004). It is defined clinically as a disorder of high blood pressure at rest. Mortality from cardiovascular disease increases progressively as BP rises from 115/75 mmHg in a linear, continuous and independent manner (COSTA *et al.*, 2013).

High blood pressure is one of the most important risk factors for the development of various cardiovascular and cerebrovascular diseases and for kidney failure. High BP is responsible for 25 and 40% of the multifactorial etiology of ischemic heart disease and strokes, respectively (FUCHS, 2004). This multiplicity of consequences places arterial hypertension at the origin of cardiovascular diseases and therefore characterizes it as one of the causes of the greatest reduction in the quality and life expectancy of individuals (Epidemiology and Health Services 2006). Cardiovascular diseases are a major public health problem and are the leading cause of death in Brazil and worldwide (CHOBANIAN *et al.*, 2003).

The correct diagnosis and classification is based on accurate BP recording, which is often incorrectly determined. When measuring BP, it is recommended that the patient should have been sitting in a stress-free environment for at least 5 minutes before the assessment, and should not have smoked, exercised or eaten in the last 30 minutes (MACPHEE and MASSIE, 2006). It is also important that the patient remains sitting up straight, with their arms resting at heart level. The cuff is placed on the brachial artery, on the upper portion of the forearm, which should cover 80% of it. It is recommended that two recordings are made and that there is a 5-minute interval between each recording (INDRIAGO, 2007).

Ambulatory blood pressure monitoring (ABPM) is better at detecting target organ damage than ambulatory measurements alone. ABPM is a non-invasive, intermittent blood pressure measurement method that allows for a large number of measurements, enabling better interpretation of the patient's blood pressure behavior throughout the day. The use of ABPM can be started 24 hours before the dental assessment with blood pressure measurements on average every 12 minutes. It can be continued during the dental appointment with blood pressure recordings every 3 minutes (SANTELLO AND AMODEO, 2004).

In 2003, the National Pressure High Blood Education Program promulgated its latest recommendations for hypertension. This seventh revision by the Joint National Committee on Prevention, Detection, Evaluation and Treatment of High Blood Pressure was known as the JNC-7 Report (CHOBANIAN et al., 2003). New guidelines are currently being presented and an updated classification is included which redefines "normal" blood pressure as < 120/80 mmHg, and a new category of pre-hypertension (120-130/8089 mmHg) has also been established, which encompasses the categories previously designated as "normal" and "borderline" hypertension (LITTLE, 2008). For the majority of the population, blood pressure should be below 140 and/or 90 mmHg, except for diabetics (<130/85 mmHg) and chronic kidney disease (up to < 120/75 mmHg) (BRAZILIAN HYPERTENSION SOCIETY, 2015).

In 2010, the Brazilian Society of Hypertension published the VI Brazilian Hypertension Guidelines, where the blood pressure limits considered normal are arbitrary. Borderline pressure is equivalent to high-normal pressure or pre-hypertension (Table 1).

Table 1- Classification of blood pressure according to casual measurement in the doctor's office according to the VI Brazilian Hypertension Guidelines (2010).

Classification		Systolic pressure
Diastolic pressure		
Great	< 120	< 80
Normal	<130	< 85
Borderline*	130-139	85-89
Stage 1 hypertension	140-159	90-99
Hypertension stage 2	160-179	100-109
Stage 3 hypertension	> 180	> 110
Isolated systolic hypertension	> 140	< 90
When systolic and diastolic pressures are in different categories, the higher one should be used to classify blood pressure.		

1High-normal pressure or pre-hypertension are terms that are equivalent in the literature
SOURCE: VI Brazilian Hypertension Guidelines, 2010.

The condition of hypertension can cause damage and even death if it is not diagnosed and controlled. Around 77% of people who have had their first stroke are hypertensive. In addition, high blood pressure increases the risk of stroke by 4 to 6 times. 75% of people with congestive heart failure (CHF) have high blood pressure, 69% with a first acute myocardial infarction (AMI) have high blood pressure and the second leading cause of chronic kidney disease is hypertension. Hypertension can also cause problems such as erectile dysfunction, dementia and loss of vision (BRAZILIAN HYPERTENSION

SOCIETY, 2015).

3.2 Etiology

BP is determined by the amount of blood the heart pumps, i.e. cardiac output, and the resistance to blood flow in the vascular system. Cardiac output, in turn, is determined by heart rate and the amount of blood ejected with each beat, i.e. stroke volume. High blood pressure, therefore, is the result of inflexible narrowed arteries, a high heart rate, increased blood volume, stronger heart contractions, or any combination of the above. The heart works in two stages: the contraction to expel blood, when the force is maximum, which is called systole, and the relaxation of the heart between heart contractions, when the force is minimal, which is called diastole The heart needs to exert pressure when pumping blood in order for it to circulate in the body. In this way, the heart contracts, in what is called systole, and pushes a large amount of blood into the arteries. This is known as systolic blood pressure (SBP). When the heart relaxes, the pressure in the blood vessels decreases; this is why it is known as diastolic blood pressure (DBP), (MENIN et al., 2006; SOCIEDADE BRASILEIRA DE HIPERTENSÂO, 2015).

In other words, when there is an increase in the volume of blood to be ejected, for example when the kidneys don't function normally or when the heart contracts insufficiently, or when the heart rate increases, i.e. the heart beats more times per minute to eject a certain volume of blood, or when the resistance offered by the arteries to the passage of blood is increased, there is an increase in blood pressure. Another possibility is that the larger caliber arteries lose their normal flexibility and become rigid, so that they cannot expand to allow the blood pumped by the heart to pass through. Thus, the blood ejected with each heartbeat is forced through a smaller space than normal and blood pressure rises. The hallmark of high blood pressure is ultimately increased vascular resistance. This can happen, for example, when very thin arteries (arterioles) temporarily contract due to nerve stimulation or hormones in the blood (SOCIEDADE BRASILEIRA DE HIPERTENSÂO, 2015).

Mean arterial pressure (MAP) is calculated by multiplying diastolic BP by two, adding systolic BP and dividing by three. Diastolic pressure is multiplied by two because, on average, the heart spends about twice as long in diastole as it does in systole (BAVITZ, 2006). The values are read by a measurement in millimeters of mercury (mmHg) (BRAZILIAN HYPERTENSION SOCIETY, 2015).

Long-term BP regulation is controlled predominantly by the kidneys through their variable release of the enzyme renin. Renin goes on to cleave angiotensinogen into angiotensin 1, which is converted by the angiotensin-converting enzyme (ACE) into angiotensin 2. Angiotensin 2 causes vasoconstriction, i.e. high vascular resistance, and stimulates the release of aldosterone, an enzyme that increases sodium reabsorption in the kidney. The increase in sodium reabsorption leads to an increase in blood volume, which results in a rise in BP. In short, during a given day or week, blood pressure readings are controlled by mainly one of the kidneys, while fear and stress can, through the autonomic nervous system, quickly and dramatically raise these values (BAVITZ, 2006).

Little et al., 2008 further describes that control mechanisms include neural reflexes and the continuous maintenance of sympathetic vasomotor tone; neurotransmitters such as norepinephrine, extracellular fluid and sodium storage; the renin-angiotensin-aldosterone pressure system; and hormones and locally active substances such as prostaglandins, kinins, adenosine and hydrogen ions (H^+). Many other factors can have an effect on blood pressure. Increased blood viscosity (e.g. polycythemia) can cause a rise in blood pressure resulting from an increase in resistance to flow. A decrease in blood volume or tissue fluid volume, such as hemorrhagic anemia, reduces BP. Conversely, an increase in blood volume or tissue fluid volume, such as sodium/liquid retention, increases BP. Increased cardiac output associated with exercise, fever and thyrotoxicosis can also trigger an increase in BP (LITTLE et al., 2008).

The determinants of blood pressure (BP) are therefore cardiac output and peripheral resistance, and any change in one or the other, or both, interferes with the maintenance of normal blood pressure levels. Several mechanisms control peripheral resistance and cardiac output: cardiac, renal, neural, hormonal, ionic, vascular and structural mechanisms, known as the physiopathogenic mechanisms of SAH. These complex mechanisms interact and balance each other, and are responsible for maintaining blood pressure as well as for its moment-to-moment variation. It is known that a dysfunction of these BP control systems results in hypertension. However, the complex interaction between these physiological systems, as well as environmental influences, such as excess salt in the diet and psycho-emotional stimuli, make it difficult to determine whether the alterations found in hypertensive patients are the primary cause of hypertension or the consequence of other as yet unknown dysfunctions (SCHAIRA, 2005).

SAH can have two origins: primary or secondary. The etiology of primary or essential hypertension, found in around 90% to 95% of patients, cannot be determined. This disease occurs due to alterations in the BP control system caused by the interaction of genetic factors with environmental factors, such as excess sodium in the diet, smoking, obesity and stress. Other patients who don't fit into this first definition are classified as having a secondary origin, which can come from other pathologies such as renal artery stenosis, pheochromocytoma, Cushing's syndrome, primary hyperaldosteronism and also the use of drugs such as alcohol, oral contraceptives, sympathomimetics, corticosteroids, cocaine and others (SCHAIRA, 2005).

In forms of secondary hypertension, representing the other 10% of patients (LITTLE, 2008), an underlying cause or condition can be identified such as renal parenchymal disease, followed by renovascular disease and various adrenal disorders (KAPLAN, 2005). Most of the conditions that cause secondary hypertension trigger a rise in diastolic and systolic blood pressure and can be treated and cured surgically (LITTLE, 2008). In the case of primary hypertension, control requires prolonged use of medication, which can affect dental treatment. These drugs can be from different pharmacological groups, and the most common ones used to treat hypertension are diuretics, selective and non-selective beta blockers, centrally acting adrenergic antagonists, calcium channel blockers, alpha adrenergic blockers, vasodilators, peripheral action sympathetic antagonists and angiotensin converting enzyme inhibitors (CARNEVALI ARAÚJO AND ARAGÁO ARAÚJO, 2001; ANDRADE, 2006).

3.3 Epidemiology

In the African region, there are still more deaths from infectious diseases than from non-communicable diseases. However, the prevalence of non-communicable diseases is increasing rapidly and is projected to be the cause of almost three quarters more deaths than those caused by maternal/perinatal communicable diseases and nutritional diseases by 2020, and by 2030, will finally overtake them as the most common causes of death. WHO projections show that non-communicable diseases will be responsible for a significantly higher total number of deaths over the next decade. Deaths from non-communicable diseases are projected to increase by 15% worldwide between 2010 and 2020 (from 44 million deaths). According to the WHO, the biggest increase will be seen in the regions of Africa, Southeast Asia and the Eastern Mediterranean, where it will be more than 20%. In contrast, the WHO estimates that there will be no increase in the European region. The regions projected to have the highest total number of deaths from non-communicable diseases in 2020 will be: Southeast Asia (10.4 million deaths) and the Western Pacific (12.3 million deaths) (The global burden of disease: 2004 update. Geneva, World Health Organization, 2008).

Globally, the total prevalence of hypertension in adults over the age of 25 was around 40% in 2008. The proportion of the world's population with high blood pressure, or uncontrolled hypertension, fell modestly between 1980 and 2008. However, because of population growth and ageing, the number of people with hypertension increased from 600 million in 1980 to almost 1 billion in 2008 (DANAEI, et al., 2008). In developing countries, the growth of the elderly population and increased longevity, associated with changes in dietary patterns and lifestyle, have a strong impact on the pattern of morbidity and mortality. In Brazil, projections by the United Nations (UN) (2002) indicate that the median age of the population will rise from 25.4 years in 2000 to 38.2 years in 2050. One of the consequences of this ageing population is an increase in the prevalence of chronic diseases, including SAH (EPIDEMIOLOGIA E SERVIAOS DE SAÚDE, 2006).

According to the WHO, the number of people with uncontrolled hypertension increased from 600 million in 1980 to almost one billion in 2008. Worldwide, high BP is estimated to cause 7.5 million deaths, and around 12.8% of all annual deaths (WHO, 2009; WHO, 2010). Population-based epidemiological studies are essential for understanding the distribution of exposure to and illness from hypertension in a given region, country or even the world, and the factors and conditions that influence the dynamics of these risk patterns in the community studied. The identification of major risk factors for cardiovascular disease, effective control strategies combined with community education and targeted monitoring of high-risk individuals have contributed to a substantial drop in mortality in almost all developed countries (REDDY AND YUSUF, 1998). Among the countries' income groups, the prevalence of high blood pressure was consistently high, with high and lower-middle income countries, lower-middle and all with rates of around 40% for both sexes. The prevalence in high-income countries was lower, at 35% for both sexes (WHO, 2010).

In all WHO regions, men have a slightly higher prevalence of high blood pressure than women, but this difference was only statistically significant in the Region of the Americas and the European Region (WHO, 2010). Pereira et. al. (2009), in a quantitative systematic review from 2003 to 2008 of 44 studies in 35 countries, revealed an overall prevalence of 37.8% in men and 32.2% in women. Still on the prevalence of high BP, there are reports of a higher prevalence in the WHO African Region, which was 46% for both genders. The lowest prevalence of high blood pressure was in the WHO Region of the Americas, with 35% for both genders (GLOBAL ATLAS ON CARDIOVASCULAR DISEASES PREVENTION AND CONTROL, 2011).

In the region of Tubarao, Santa Catarina, Brazil, Pereira et al. (2007) aimed to estimate the prevalence, knowledge, treatment and control of systemic arterial hypertension in the urban adult population. To achieve the study's objective, they used energy consumption data to compose the sample in strata to ensure socio-economic representativeness of the population, where there was an association between *per capita* energy consumption and family income. They observed a high estimated prevalence of hypertension (36.4%), a low level of ignorance (55.6%), and a low level of treatment (46.8%) and optimal control of the disease (10.1%), emphasizing the need for preventive measures in Tubarao - SC. In another review article, Passos et al., 2006, analyzed population-based studies on the prevalence of hypertension in adults in Brazil from 1990 onwards. In the 13 studies selected, they found that prevalence rates showed that around 20% of adults had hypertension, without distinguishing between sexes, but also with a clear upward trend with age. However, it is worth noting that these studies were restricted to the South and Southeast regions (PASSOS et al., 2006).

Population surveys in Brazilian cities over the last 20 years have indicated a prevalence of SAH of over 30% (CESARINO *et al.*, 2008; ROSÁRIO *et al.,* 2009). Considering BP values > 140/90 mmHg, 22 studies found a prevalence of between 22.3% and 43.9% (average 32.5%), with more than 50% between 60 and 69 years old and 75% over 70 years old (ROSÁRIO *et al.*, 2009). In this context, NEDER and

BORGES, 2006, surveyed the studies described above, which estimate the prevalence of SAH in Brazil, in an attempt to evaluate these surveys and their veracity and agreement.

SAH is the most important risk factor for the development of cardiovascular, cerebrovascular and renal diseases, being responsible for at least 40% of deaths from stroke, 25% of deaths from coronary artery disease and, in combination with diabetes, 50% of cases of end-stage renal failure. With the current criteria for diagnosing hypertension (BP 140/90 mmHg), the prevalence in the urban adult Brazilian population varies from 22.3% to 43.9%, depending on the city assessed. The main importance of identifying and controlling hypertension lies in reducing its complications, such as cerebrovascular disease, coronary artery disease, heart failure, chronic kidney disease and peripheral artery disease (PASSOS; ASSIS; BARRETO, 2006). Heart disease is one of the main consequences of SAH and it is estimated that 20 million Americans are now living with some aspect of this disease (LIFSHE, 2004).

According to the 2015 Heart Disease and Stroke Statistics study by the American Heart Association, during the last decade surveyed, from 2001 to 2011, the death rate from hypertension in more than 190 countries surveyed increased by 13.2% (Figure 1). Brazil, for its part, ranks sixth among the countries with the highest death rate from heart disease, heart attacks and hypertension among men and women aged 35 to 74. In detail, Russia is in first place with 1,639 (out of 100,000 surveyed), Brazil in sixth place with 552 and the United States in tenth place with 352 (BRAZILIAN HYPERTENSION SOCIETY, 2015).

According to a survey by the World Health Organization (WHO) (2010), SAH is responsible for 9.4 million deaths worldwide and affects 30% of the adult Brazilian population, reaching more than 50% in the elderly and is present in 5% of children and adolescents in Brazil, according to estimates by the SBH (BRAZILIAN SOCIETY OF HYPERTENSION, 2015).

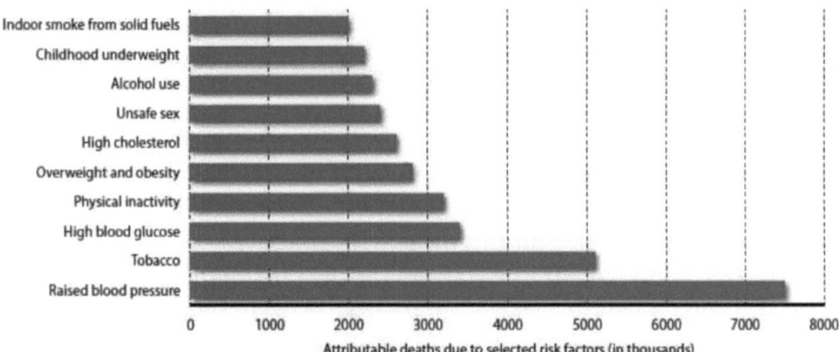

Figure 1. Ranking of 10 selected risk factors for causes of death. Source: Global Atlas on Cardiovascular Diseases Prevention and Control (2011).

3.4 Diagnosis and Classification

The demarcation line that defines SAH considers systolic BP values > 140 mmHg and/or diastolic BP > 90mmHg in office measurements. Repeated blood pressure measurements under ideal conditions are recommended for the diagnosis to be validated, i.e. on at least 3 occasions (FIGUEREDO *et al.*, 2009).

Different possibilities for classifying BP behavior in terms of diagnosis are considered, according to the new forms of definition: true normotension, isolated systolic hypertension, white coat hypertension and masked hypertension (VI BRAZILIAN HYPERTENSION GUIDELINES, 2010).

3.4.1 - True normotension

True normotension is considered to be when office measurements are in the normal range, provided that all the conditions laid down in these guidelines are met (Table 1), with regard to pressure being considered optimal with values <120 (systolic) and < 80 (diastolic) up to a borderline pressure of values between 130-139 (systolic) and 85-89 (diastolic). In addition, you should consider average blood pressures from Self-Measured Blood Pressure (SMABP) or Home Blood Pressure Monitoring (HBPM), or even in the waking period from ABPM < 130 x 85 mmHg (MANCIA *et al.*, 1995).

3.4.2 - Isolated systolic hypertension

Isolated systolic hypertension is defined as abnormal systolic BP behavior with normal diastolic BP. This described hypertension and pulse pressure are important risk factors for cardiovascular disease in middle-aged and elderly patients (GUS, 2009).

3.4.3 - White coat hypertension

HBP is defined when the patient has persistently high BP measurements (> 140/90 mmHg) in the doctor's office and BP averages considered normal either at home, by AMPA or MRPA, or by ABPM (MANCIA, et al., 1995);

PARATI et al., 2008). Available evidence points to a worse cardiovascular prognosis for HBP compared to normotensive patients (MANCIA et al., 2006). Up to 70% of patients with this BP behavior will have hypertension by ABPM and/or ABPM over a ten-year period (MANCIA et al., 1995).

3.4.4 - Masked hypertension

It is defined as the clinical situation characterized by normal BP values in the doctor's office (< 140/90 mmHg), but with elevated BP by ABPM during the waking period or in MRPA. Patients with masked hypertension (MH) should be identified and monitored, as they are at risk of developing target organ damage in a similar way to hypertensive patients (DE GREEFF, 2010).

3.6 Clinical presentation

3.6.1 Signs and symptoms

SAH can be considered a silent disease, asymptomatic for several years. In many cases, the only sign is high blood pressure.

The earliest sign of hypertension is the measurement of high blood pressure; however, fundoscopic examination of the eyes can show early changes due to hypertension, consisting of narrowed arterioles with sclerosis. Even if hypertension remains asymptomatic for years, when symptoms occur, they include headache, ringing in the ears and dizziness (LITTLE, et al., 2008). These symptoms, however, are non-specific to hypertension and can often be observed in the same way in normotensive individuals (KAPLAN, 2005).

3.6.2 Laboratory findings

The Seventh Report of the Joint National Committee on Prevention, Detection, Evaluation and Treatment of Hypertension (JNC 7) recommends that patients with persistent hypertension should have routine laboratory tests, including a 12-lead electrocardiogram, urinalysis, blood glucose, hematocrit, and serum potassium, creatinine, calcium and lipid profile. Doctors need these baseline laboratory values before starting drug therapy (LITTLE et al., 2008). Complementary assessment is aimed at detecting clinical or subclinical lesions in order to better stratify cardiovascular risk. In the presence of elements indicative of cardiovascular disease and associated diseases, in patients with two or more risk factors, and in patients over 40 years of age with diabetes, the following complementary tests are indicated: chest X-ray, echocardiogram, microalbuminuria, carotid ultrasound, exercise test, glycated hemoglobin, ABPM, ABPM. Other tests such as pulse wave velocity may be indicated to complement the diagnosis. An investigation into secondary hypertension is indicated when there is suspicion from the history, physical examination or initial laboratory assessment (MANCIA et al., 2007; BRAZILIAN HYPERTENSION SOCIETY, 2015).

3.6.3 Hypertension and associated medical conditions

Undetected and uncontrolled hypertension, which increases cardiovascular risk, is one of the main contributors to stroke worldwide (WHO, 2010). BP levels have been shown to be positively and progressively related to the risk of stroke and coronary heart disease. In some age groups, the risk of CVD doubles with each incremental increase of 20/10 mmHg in blood pressure, starting as low as 115/75 mmHg (GLOBAL ATLAS ON CARDIOVASCULAR DISEASES PREVENTION AND CONTROL 2011). There are reports in the literature that undetected and uncontrolled hypertension, which increases cardiovascular risk, is one of the main contributors to stroke worldwide (DANAEI et al., 2011).

In addition to coronary heart disease and cerebral vascular disease, uncontrolled blood pressure causes heart failure, kidney failure, peripheral vascular disease and damage to retinal blood vessels and visual impairment (KAPLAN, 2005).

Severe hypertension, defined as BP > 180/ 120, can be classified as an urgency or emergency (NATIONAL HEART LUNG AND BLOOD INSTITUTE, 2004). Hypertensive emergencies are characterized by a severe rise in blood pressure with evidence of imminent or progressive dysfunction in certain target organs (heart, brain, vessels and kidneys), such as hypertensive encephalopathy, intercerebral haemorrhage, stroke, renal failure, acute MI, left ventricular failure with pulmonary oedema or unstable angina *pectoris*. Patients need immediate blood pressure reduction (within 1 hour) and should be referred immediately to an intensive care unit (ICU) (RIDKER and LIBBY, 2005). These same patients, but with adverse symptoms such as headache, shortness of breath, epistaxis or anxiety, require urgent treatment, but do not constitute an emergency. Such patients are characterized as non-cooperators, i.e. they do not adhere to drug treatment or are inadequately medicated. They should receive treatment as soon as possible to control BP, initially including the administration of short-acting oral antihypertensive medication, followed by a few hours of observation and subsequent adjustments to medication. However, these patients should not show evidence of an association with progressive damage to target organs (LITTLE et al., 2008).

3.6.4 Non-drug and drug treatment

Maintaining systolic and diastolic blood pressure below 140/90 mmHg is associated with a reduction in cardiovascular complications (WHO, 2007). The risk of stroke and acute myocardial infarction in people with high cardiovascular impairment and/or high blood pressure can be reduced through non-pharmacological and pharmacological measures (WHO, 2010). A dietary approach plan for hypertension has been well studied, which recommends eating fruit, vegetables and low-fat dairy products, combined with sodium restriction to less than 2.4 g per day (BAVITZ, 2006). The main non-drug recommendations for primary prevention of hypertension are: healthy eating, controlled consumption of sodium and alcohol, potassium intake, combating sedentary lifestyles and smoking, and lifestyle changes (weight loss, physical activity). The aim of this complementary therapy is to maintain blood pressure levels below 140/90 mmHg, with a consequent reduction in cardiovascular complications. In hypertensive and diabetic patients and/or those with kidney disease, the goal is to achieve even lower values (130/80 mmHg) (CHOBANIAN et al., 2003). These measures are very important for people with diabetes, as they are particularly vulnerable to heart attacks and strokes (GLOBAL ATLAS ON CARDIOVASCULAR DISEASES PREVENTION AND CONTROL, 2011).

These lifestyle modifications are often inexpensive and have few contraindications and/or adverse effects (BAVITZ, 2006). The recommended time period for lifestyle modification measures alone in hypertensive patients and those with borderline blood pressure behavior and low cardiovascular risk is a maximum of six months. If patients are not responding to these measures after three months, a new assessment should be made in six months to confirm BP control (BRAZILIAN SOCIETY OF HYPERTENSION, 2015). Even so, many people are unable to achieve desirable BP levels with these modifications and are therefore prescribed drugs in combination to keep their BP within the therapeutic range (BAVITZ, 2006).

In patients at medium, high or very high risk, regardless of BP, the approach should be combined (non-drug and drug) in order to reach the recommended target as early as possible (BRAZILIAN SOCIETY OF HYPERTENSION, 2015).

Studies have been carried out to evaluate the efficacy and safety of drugs in the prevention of SAH. In the TROPHY (WILLIAMS *et al.*, 2008) and PHARAO (LÜDERS *et al.*, 2008) studies, the drug strategy was well tolerated and prevented the development of hypertension in young, high-risk populations. For the management of individuals with borderline BP behavior, it is recommended to consider drug treatment only in conditions of high or very high overall cardiovascular risk. To date, no study has had sufficient power to indicate drug treatment for individuals with borderline BP without evidence of cardiovascular disease. The therapeutic decision should be based on cardiovascular risk, considering the presence of risk factors, target organ damage and/or established cardiovascular disease, and not just on the level of BP (VI BRAZILIAN HYPERTENSION GUIDELINES, 2010).

The implementation of preventive measures for SAH is still a major challenge for health professionals and managers. In Brazil, around 75% of the population's health care is provided by the public Unified Health System - SUS, while the Complementary Health System assists around 46.5 million. Primary prevention and early detection are the most effective ways of avoiding disease and should be priority goals for health professionals (VI DIRETRIZES BRASILEIRAS DE HIPERTENSÁO, 2010).

The population's access to primary care for cardiovascular risk assessment and essential drugs for reducing cardiovascular risk can improve the health outcomes of people with hypertension (WHO, 2010).

3.6.5 Antihypertensives (drug interactions and adverse effects)

All patients with diagnosed hypertension should be treated with the aim, for most hypertensive patients, of reducing blood pressure to <140/90mmHg. However, for patients with hypertension associated with diabetes or kidney disease, the value to be achieved should be <130/80mmHg. Evidence shows the clear benefits of aggressive treatment for hypertension (LITTLE et al., 2008).

Many drugs are currently available for the treatment of hypertension (LITTLE et al., 2008). For most patients, the first drug administered to treat high blood pressure is a diuretic. Diuretics (hydrochlorothiazide, triamterene, furosemide) are the most researched class of drugs and work to reduce BP both by decreasing vascular resistance and reducing blood volume (BAVITZ, 2006).

Beta-blockers (propranolol, sotolol) are also often prescribed to lower BP by reducing the speed and strength of contractions. They are often used in patients with co-existing heart problems, such as angina and a history of myocardial infarction. Selective beta-blockers (atenolol, metoprolol) preferentially target and block beta-1 receptors on the heart, avoiding beta-2 receptors in the bronchioles. These receptors in the bronchioles react to sympathetic stimulation by relaxing the smooth muscles, generating bronchodilation. Non-selective beta-blockers are therefore contraindicated in asthma patients, as asthma patients who usually use their inhalers (beta agonists) will have their action "blocked" by their antihypertensive medication (BAVITZ, 2006).

ACE inhibitors (captopril, enalapril) act by slowing down the renin angiotensin system. They produce vasodilation by interfering with the conversion of angiotensin 1 into angiotensin 2. By reducing angiotensin 2, vasoconstriction and BP reduction decrease. In the case of calcium channel blockers (amlodipine, nifedipine, diltiazem) they typically reduce all variables in BP, minimizing the influx of calcium into smooth and cardiac muscle. They decrease total peripheral resistance and often slow the heart rate and decrease the force of contraction.

Alpha-blocking agents (prazosin, terazosin) prevent norepinephrine (the sympathetic transmitter) from binding to receptors in the arterioles, immediately leading to vasodilation. Other direct-acting vasodilators (nitroglycerin, minoxidil) work independently of the ANS to relax the vascular smooth muscle. Some agents (methyldopa, clonidine) act on the CNS to reduce sympathetic nervous system action (BAVITZ, 2006).

A relatively new class of drugs is the angiotensin 2 receptor blockers (e.g. losartan, telmisartan), which work to prevent the restriction promoted by vasoconstriction by binding to smooth muscle sites in the arterial pathways, thus aiming to promote vasodilation (BAVITZ, 2006).

Most of the existing drugs in each class of antihypertensive have their own adverse effects. Some adverse effects deserve special attention. Gingival hyperplasia can be seen with the use of most calcium channel blocking drugs (LITTLE et al., 2008), with an incidence of 1.7% to 38% (HERMAN et al., 2004). Nifedipine is the most notorious, and while surgery can temporarily reduce bleeding in painful gums, cessation of the drug is usually necessary for healing (BAVITZ, 2006). Mercurial diuretics can cause allergic or toxic oral lesions (LITTLE et al., 2008). The dentist should communicate with the doctor to switch to another class of antihypertensive drug (BAVITZ, 2006; COSTA et al., 2013).

There are reports that patients with severe hypertension tend to bleed excessively after surgical procedures or trauma, however, excessive bleeding in hypertensive patients is not common and is a controversial observation. ACE inhibitors can cause neutropenia, resulting in delayed healing or bleeding gums. Non-allergic angioedema can be caused by ACE inhibitors. Mouth burning has also been linked to the use of ACE inhibitors (LITTLE et al., 2008).

Xerostomia, on the other hand, is another side effect that is common to practically all patients who use antihypertensive drugs, especially diuretics (INDRIAGO, 2007; LITTLE et al., 2008). Patients who take more than one drug in combination are more seriously affected. Examples of the known complications of xerostomia as a result of drug administration are numerous, ranging from dry mouth sensation, cervical caries, tongue burning, decreased retention of removable dentures and even difficulty chewing and swallowing (CORRÉA et al., 2005; HERMAN et al., 2004). Treatment involves topical fluoride application and possibly systemic drugs such as pilocarpine or cevimeline. Many patients simply get into the habit of swishing their mouths with water and chewing sugar-free gum. These are simple but effective solutions (INDRIAGO, 2007). Dentists should also advise their patients to avoid mouthwashes containing alcohol, as these can exacerbate dry mouth (BAVITZ, 2006).

Lichenoid reactions, a condition clinically indistinguishable from lichen planus, can occur from many antihypertensive drugs and have been reported with the use of thiazide drugs, methyldopa, propranolol and lebetalol (BAVITZ, 2006; LITTLE et al., 2008). Changing the antihypertensive drug can help, but a biopsy is indicated if the lesions do not regress. Treatment for lichenoid lesions is only necessary if they become symptomatic. High-potency steroids such as clobetasol or the antimetabolite cyclosporine are both generally effective (CONROTTO, et al., 2006).

Cases of orthostatic hypotension occur to varying degrees in all patients who have to use anti-hypertensive drugs. Healthcare professionals, such as dentists, are encouraged to slowly return patients to an upright position after dental care, and to have them sit on the edge of the chair for 30 to 60 seconds before standing up. Another precaution cited in JNC7 involves the interaction between antihypertensive drugs and general anesthetic agents (BAVITZ, 2006).

Finally, there is interaction between non-steroidal anti-inflammatory drugs and antihypertensive agents, but it only begins to occur after 2 to 3 weeks of daily use of non-steroidal anti-inflammatory drugs. Indomethacin seems to be the non-steroidal anti-inflammatory drug most likely to reduce the effectiveness of antihypertensive medication (BAVITZ, 2006).

3.7 Dental treatment

According to ARSATI et al. (2010) hypertension is the fourth most frequent medical condition in the dental clinic. In this context, the dental surgeon plays an important role in the possible diagnosis of these patients, most of whom are unaware that they have hypertension because it is an asymptomatic disease. If this is suspected, it is essential to refer them to a medical service to confirm the diagnosis and start treatment (COSTA, et al., 2013). Patients who have not been diagnosed with hypertension, but who have high blood pressure, should be warned that their BP is high and should be encouraged to see their doctor (LITTLE et al., 2008).

The clinical history obtained at the first consultation should include the diagnosis of hypertension, form of treatment, identification of antihypertensive drugs, the patient's adherence to the therapeutic regimen, the presence of symptoms associated with hypertension, risk factors, indications of secondary hypertension and target organ damage, socio-economic aspects and characteristics of the patient's lifestyle, previous or current consumption of medications or drugs that may interfere with their treatment (anti-inflammatory drugs, anorexiants, nasal decongestants, etc.) and the level of stability of the disease (LITTLE et al., 2008; BRAZILIAN SOCIETY OF HYPERTENSION, 2015). In addition to taking an anamnesis, all patients should have their blood pressure measured, which should be carried out as a routine procedure for all new patients and at return visits. At the first assessment, measurements should be taken on both sides of the body. If there is a difference, the arm with the highest value should always be used as a reference for subsequent measurements. At least three measurements should be taken at each visit, with a suggested interval of one minute between them, although this is controversial. The average of the last two measurements should be considered the real BP. If the systolic and/or diastolic pressures obtained show a difference of more than 4 mmHg, new measurements should be taken until a lower difference is obtained. The recommended position for measuring blood pressure is sitting. Measurements in the orthostatic and supine positions should be taken at least at the first assessment in all individuals and at every assessment in the elderly, diabetics, people with autonomic disorders, alcoholics and/or those taking antihypertensive medication (BRAZILIAN HYPERTENSION SOCIETY, 2015) (Figure 1).

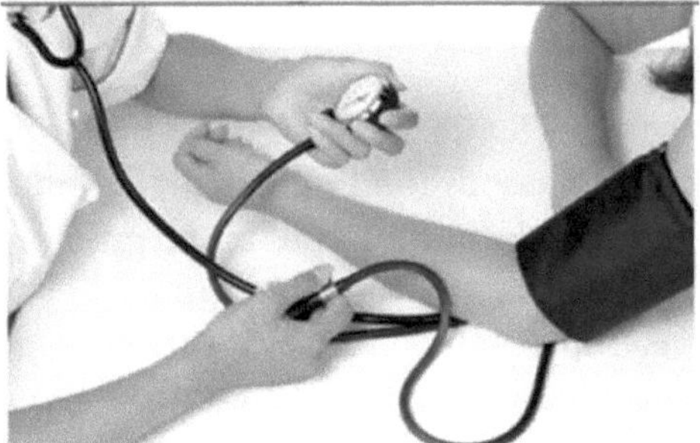

Figure 2. Taking blood pressure. Check correct position of patient and cuff.
SOURCE: Google images.

More frequent BP measurements are indicated for patients who are not committed to treatment, whose pressure is not adequately controlled or who have comorbid conditions such as heart failure, previous MI or stroke. If a patient with BP above the stage 2 level is treated, the blood pressure cuff should be left on the patient's arm during the consultation and checked periodically (LITTLE, et al., 2008).

The individual should be referred by the health professional for specialized medical investigation for arterial diseases if they present pressure differences between the upper limbs greater than 20/10 mmHg for the systolic/diastolic pressures respectively (BRAZILIAN HYPERTENSION SOCIETY, 2015). However, dentists in particular must be able to treat patients with hypertension and must be able to make treatment safe, appropriate and effective with full consideration of the patient's heart condition, which is often a cause of hypertension. Considering that cardiac patients often have more than one category of disease, it is suggested that they be assessed separately for a clearer understanding of the extent and involvement of the disease (NYSDJ, 2004).

The American Society of Anesthesiologists (ASA) physical classification system has been used since 1941 to help assess the risk and potential complications that can occur in the dental office, for example. The higher the ASA class (I to IV), the greater the risk to the patient from both a surgical and anesthetic point of view (FLEISCHER, 2004).

TABLE 1- American Society of Anesthesiologists (ASA) physical classification system.

ASA CLASS	DEFINITION
ASA class I	A normal healthy patient
ASA class II	A patient with mild systemic disease
ASA class III	A patient with severe systemic disease
ASA Class IV	A dying patient who is not expected to survive surgery

SOURCE: FLEISCHER, 2004.

The prudent dentist may choose not to perform elective care on an ASA Class III patient whose BP is 175/105. Classifying a patient in ASA I to IV, however, is subjective, even for doctors, which has led many to look for alternative risk assessment strategies (BAVITZ, 2006).

The American College of Cardiology and the American Heart Association have published practical guidelines for the pre-operative assessment of patients with various types of cardiovascular disease who are undergoing non-cardiac surgery, which can be used to help answer questions about the risk of a serious event such as stroke and MI. Periodontal and oral and maxillofacial surgery fit into this context of non-cardiac surgery, so these guidelines are directly applicable to this type of procedure. Determining risk includes assessing three factors: the risk imposed by the patient's cardiovascular disease, the risk imposed by the surgery or procedure to be performed, and the risk imposed by the patient's functional cardiopulmonary reserve or capacity (EAGLE et al.,

2002). The risk imposed by the presence of a specific cardiovascular condition or disease is stratified into higher, intermediate and lower risks of an unfavorable event occurring intraoperatively. The JNC 7 recommendation of immediate treatment for patients with blood pressure >180/110 is taken into account. The risk imposed by the type of surgery (or procedure) is also stratified into high (risk >5%) and low (<1%). Superficial surgical procedures, which include minor oral surgery and periodontal surgery and non-surgical dental procedures, are classified as low risk. The third factor involved in risk assessment is the determination of the patient's functional or reserve cardiopulmonary capacity, defined as metabolic equivalents (METs) (LITTLE et al., 2008).

The METS concept is being used for a concrete assessment. A MET is defined as 3.5 mL O2/kg/min, (EAGLE et al., 2002; STEINHAUER et al., 2005). Essentially it is a test of the patient's ability to perform physical work, with the following examples: 1 to 4 METS - eating, dressing, walking around the house, washing dishes; 4 to 10 METS - climbing at least one flight of stairs, walking on flat ground at 6.4 km/h, running short distances, playing golf; R10 METS - swimming, playing tennis or soccer. People with abilities of 4 METS or less are at high risk of medical complications. Patients who can perform 10 METS or more are at very low risk. In the case of anxious patients who have a BP of 200/115mmHg, but can perform 10 METS of work, they would probably not have any complications during a simple extraction procedure (BAVITZ, 2006).

The main concern when carrying out dental treatment on a patient with hypertension is the possibility that, during the course of treatment, the patient may experience an acute rise in blood pressure, which could trigger serious consequences such as stroke or MI. This acute rise in BP can result from the release of endogenous catecholamines in response to stress and anxiety, the injection of exogenous catecholamines in the form of vasoconstrictors in the local anesthetic, or the absorption of a vasoconstrictor from the gum retraction thread. Other concerns include possible drug interactions between the patient's antihypertensive medications and the prescribed medications, as well as oral adverse effects that can be caused by antihypertensive medications, already mentioned in a previous topic and specified in the table below (LITTLE, et al., 2008) (TABLE 2).

Table 2 - Drug interaction with antihypertensive agents.

Drugs	Interaction drugs	Effects
Diuretics	NSAIDs	Effect of anti-hypertensive decreases
Diuretics	Barbiturates	Orthostatic hypertension
Diuretics	Fluconazole	High levels of Floconazole
Beta blockers	NSAIDs	Decrease in anti-inflammatory effect hypertensive
Beta blockers (non-selective)	Epinephrine	Elevations BP transients
Beta blockers Beta blockers	Local anesthetics	Decrease in the rate of amide metabolism Decrease in
(non-selective)	Bronchodilators	Response to inhaled bronchodilator
ACE inhibitors	NSAIDs	Effect of anti-hypertensive decreases
Calcium channel blockers	Benzodiazepines	Increased sedation
Calcium channel blockers	parenteral anesthetic agents	Intraoperative hypertension
Calcium channel blockers	Aspirin	Increased anti-hypertensive effect
Calcium channel blockers	NSAIDs	Decreased anti-hypertensive effect
Blockers Alpha	NSAIDs	Decreased anti-hypertensive effect
Blockers Alpha	CNS depressants	Anti increased hypertension

Direct-acting vasodilators	NSAIDs	Decreased anti-hypertensive effect
Direct-acting vasodilators	Opioids	Increased anti-hypertensive effect
Central action agents	Epinephrine	Transient rise in BP
Central action agents	NSAIDs	Anti decreased hypertension
Central action agents	Sedatives	Increased sedative effect
Central action agents	Opiods	Increased anti-hypertensive effect
Angiotensin 2 blocker receiver	Systemic antifungals	Increased anti-hypertensive effect
Angiotensin receptor blocker	2 Sedatives of	Anti-effect increased hypertension

Abbreviations: CNS, central nervous system; NSAIDs, non-steroidal anti-inflammatory drugs.
Source: BAVITZ, 2006.

The literature highlights studies on the ability of epinephrine to react with various antihypertensive agents and other classes of drugs to potentially produce cardiovascular complications. In summary, these are mainly epinephrine/non-selective beta-blockers can cause hypertension, and a reflex bradycardia are potential consequences of this drug combination; epinephrine/diuretics often produce hypocalcemia which is aggravated by the use of adrenaline, as well as low potassium levels in the blood, which increases the risk of arrhythmias; and the epinephrine/cocaine combination, indicating that any suspicion of cocaine use should alert the dentist to use epinephrine with extreme caution. These last two drugs together often result in blood pressure spikes and fatal arrhythmias. Avoiding any dental care for 24 hours after suspected cocaine use is rational (HERMAN et al., 2004; MALAMED, 2004; BAVITZ, 2006).

Some hypertensive patients respond to severe psychological stress (such as anesthesia for a dental procedure) first by activating the sympathetic arm of the central nervous system, but then have an exaggerated parasympathetic response. The system's acetylcholine transmitter causes the parasympathetic of the heart to slow down, leading to a dramatic drop in BP and a resulting syncope event, such as fainting. These patients usually regain consciousness after being placed in a supine position (DEPARTMENT OF SURGICAL SPECIALTIES, 2006), a strategy that can be used in the dental field.

Many of these hypertensive patients who are also anxious respond with favorable BP to simple relaxation techniques through relaxing sounds, smells, lighting, colors, and the perception that the dentist is competent and skilled in attending to them can positively affect anxiety and BP (BAVITZ, 2006). Mishima et al., (2004), noted how the pleasant sounds of water decreased PA while the patient, on the other hand, the sounds of a dental turbine increased readings. This study also non-invasively investigated cerebral blood flow and metabolism, concluding that both changed favorably only in response to auditory stimulation. The treatment of anxiety requires a different technique, with which fear is eliminated or reduced through a significant relearning process that is the result of interactions initiated by the dentist for this purpose. This technique, called iatrosedagogy, is defined as the act of bringing calm through the behavior of the doctor or dentist performing the treatment. Two main categories are described as the iatroeducational interview and the iatroeducational clinical encounter. The iatrosedative interview is designed to initiate fear reduction through a relearning process. It is brief and economical, usually lasting no more than 10 minutes. The clinical encounter continues the process, thus lowering the level of fear at the time of care through methods such as eye contact, facial expression, vocal characteristics and body language aimed at bringing the patient closer to the professional (FRIEDMAN, 1967). Friedman and Wood (1998) pointed out that an iatrosedative interview is more effective than a standard dental interview in reducing anxiety.

Certainly, such a relaxing technique has a favorable effect on BP for some patients, but not all. Others may respond to anxiolytics, pharmacological measures such as the use of nitrous oxide or orally administered sedatives, techniques available to most general dentists. Grossman et al. in 2005 evaluated the treatment of hypertensive patients with 5 mg of diazepam compared to the ACE inhibitor captopril. The patients in this study initially presented to the emergency room with BP readings over 190/100 and responded equally well to both treatments, reducing their systolic blood pressure by an average of 30 mm Hg and diastolic values by 25 mm Hg. It should be noted, however, that pharmacotherapy does not reduce or eliminate fear, but only temporarily circumvents it. It is mainly the possibility of carrying out dental treatment that is accessible to the patient, reducing awareness and producing a temporary state of tranquillity (FRIEDMAN, 1967). An effective approach is oral premedication with short-acting benzodiazepines, such as triazolam, with one dose prescribed the night before and another dose one hour before the dental appointment. The dose is determined by the age and size of the patient and the guidelines for the selected agent (LITTLE et al., 2008). In cases where, however, pharmacological interventions such as anxiolytics are not available or if they fail to bring the patient's BP down, the doctor in charge can be contacted to advise on treatment (BAVITZ, 2006). However, Malamed (2004) makes it clear that the responsibility for treatment rests solely in the hands of the person carrying out the treatment, and not the person advising.

Several pieces of clinical and experimental evidence suggest that OSAHS is related to the development of hypertension independently of obesity (SOCIEDADE BRASILEIRA DE HIPERTENSÂO, 2015). The combination of this and other evidence led it to be included as a cause of SAH in 2003 (SJÔSTRÔM et al., 2002). Sleep apnea is now a frequently diagnosed condition characterized by partial or complete obstruction of the upper airway during sleep. This leads to less restful sleep and daytime drowsiness, and contributes to the development of hypertension (BAVITZ, 2006). Oral appliances that move the jaw forward during sleep can help some patients with obstructive sleep apnea (BARCLAY AND VEGA, 2006).

3.8 Modifications to the treatment plan

An accurate preoperative assessment of the nature and severity of the patient's illness (for the purposes of risk assessment during dental treatment) can usually be determined by a careful medical history and an evaluation of the signs and symptoms of the illness. This knowledge, together with a medical consultation, if indicated, in order to clarify some basic aspects of the disease, will also facilitate communication between the dentist and doctor, and thus result in improved care.

Patients whose BP is <180/110, i.e. patients in stages 1 and 2, can receive any dental treatment indicated. However, those with high BP (above stage 2) should be assessed for the type of procedure, its duration, as well as signs and symptoms, which should be observed in order to decide whether it is better to delay elective treatment and encourage the patient to see a doctor. If it is decided to carry out the procedure, after a dental assessment, intra-operative BP monitoring in the dental chair should be considered. No elective dental procedure should be carried out on patients with uncontrolled or severe hypertension (>180/110) (AUBERTIN, 2004; LITTLE et al., 2008; RILEY AND TEREZHALMY, 2001)(Table 2). Andrade (2014) adds that it is advisable to avoid dental care for patients with uncontrolled SAH due to the risk of hypertensive crises in dental practices.

Table 3 -Dental treatment and recommendations for monitoring based on BP.

Blood pressure	Recommendation of dental treatment	Referral to a doctor
<120/80	Whatever you need	No
>120/80 but 140/90	Whatever you need	Encourage the patient to visit the doctor
>140/90 but 160/100	Whatever you need	Encourage the patient to visit the doctor
>160/100 but	Whatever it takes;	Encourage the patient to
<180/110	consider intra-operative monitoring of blood pressure classified above stage 2	visit the doctor promptly (within 1 month)
>180/110	Delaying elective treatment	Refer to a doctor as soon as possible; if the patient is symptomatic, refer immediately

SOURCE: LITTLE et al., 2008.

In patients with cardiovascular diseases such as SAH, the dental surgeon must take into account the precautions related to the use of local anesthetic solutions with vasoconstrictors, as their incorrect use can aggravate the patient's hypertension (OLIVEIRA et al., 2010). Knowledge of the patient's general health conditions is necessary through a well-conducted anamnesis, physical examination and contact with the doctor responsible for the patient, when necessary, which are fundamental for a correct diagnosis and appropriate therapy (GLICK, 2004; SHCAIRA, 2005).

Stress management for patients with hypertension is extremely important in order to reduce the chances of endogenous release of ketacolamines during the consultation. It is recommended to avoid long, stressful appointments. Short appointments in the morning seem to be better tolerated. If the patient becomes anxious or apprehensive during the appointment or if the BP rises above 179/109, the appointment can be terminated and the patient rescheduled for another day.

To aid local anesthesia, vasoconstrictors are used in conjunction with local anesthetics, which have great advantages in achieving effective anesthesia. Local anesthetics are divided into two groups: the adrenergic ones, which are: epinephrine/adrenaline, norepinephrine/noradrenaline, phenylephrine and levonordephrine, and the non-adrenergic ones such as felipressin, which is a synthetic analog of vasopressin (a hormone released by the anterior pituitary gland) (MALAMED, 2013). Local anesthesia in patients with cardiovascular problems must be efficient enough to provide effective pain control during and immediately after treatment, thus avoiding the increased secretion of catecholamines and its consequences, since a stressed patient can release up to 40 times their baseline level of catecholamines (Knoll-Kohler et al., 1989). Good local anesthesia does not normally occur with local anesthetic solutions without vasoconstrictors, and dental surgeons should opt for anesthetics with vasoconstrictors whenever possible, following certain precautions. The increase in blood pressure in patients undergoing dental treatment with the use of local anesthetics associated with adrenaline is greater in hypertensive patients than in normotensive patients. Blood pressure changes in hypertensive patients during dental treatment occur due to the use of catecholamines such as adrenaline, suggesting that felipressin, a non-sympathomimetic substance, is the vasoconstrictor of choice in these patients (COSTA et al., 2013). This issue of using local anesthetics with or without vasoconstrictors is much debated, since this procedure can further increase the patient's blood pressure, but Silvestre et al. (2011) in their study observed no hemodynamic changes between the groups that used vasoconstrictors and those that did not. Indriago (2007), on the other hand, disagrees on the use of anesthetics with vasoconstrictors, such as epinephrine, norepinephrine and felipressin. Santos et al. (2009) adds that the use of local anesthetics with vasoconstrictors is not contraindicated, as long as no more than two vials are administered per clinical session. Thus, based on the existing evidence, it seems that one or more than two tubes of 2% lidocaine with epinephrine 1:100,000 are of little clinical importance for the majority of hypertensive patients, the benefits of their use far outweighing any possible disadvantages or risks. The use of a larger amount can be well tolerated, but there is an increased risk of hemodynamic alterations (LITTLE et al., 2008). When the principles of local anesthetic technique are respected (slow injection preceded by prior aspiration) and the maximum amounts of anesthetics per session, associated with vasoconstrictors in minimal concentrations (adrenaline 1:100,000 or 1:200,000 or felipressin 0.03 IU/ml), pain control is practically guaranteed and an exaggerated response to stress is avoided (COSTA et al., 2013). It has been described that the use of epinephrine is not really recommended for patients with uncontrolled or severe hypertension and, in fact, elective dental treatment should be postponed. Anesthetics with norepinephrine and levonordefrin as vasoconstrictors should be avoided in hypertensive patients, due to the significant increase in blood pressure that these drugs cause (INDRIADO, 2007). In cases where the use of vasoconstrictors is absolutely contraindicated, anesthetic solutions based on mepivacaine 3% without vasoconstrictor can be chosen, which provide pulp anesthesia for up to 20 minutes in infiltrative injections and up to 30 to 40 minutes in regional blocks (COSTA, et al., 2013).

It is reported that in addition to the possibility of BP changes depending on the anesthetic used and the type of vasoconstrictor administered, individual factors such as a low pain threshold, poor previous dental experience and, above all, anxiety about dental treatment should be taken into account (BRAND, 1999). Peet, in 1988, evaluated the use of antihypertensive drugs from the beta-blocker class in anxious patients, concluding that these drugs reduce the release of endogenous adrenaline and can be used to treat anxiety, regardless of its cause, by reducing catecholamines in the nerve synapses.

High BP during surgery leads to increased intraoperative bleeding. While bleeding may not be of importance during restorative dentistry, it is during oral surgery. In the context of dentists operating in the office under local anesthesia, intentional reduction in BP is not feasible, such as a Le Fort osteotomy where the oral and maxillofacial specialists ask the anesthesiologists for a lower BP for the procedures (BAVITZ, 2006). In the office, appropriate precautions should be taken if aggressive oral surgery, such as multiple extractions with alveoloplasty, is planned, associated with a high BP. Special attention should also be paid to patients taking anticoagulants such as aspirin or warfarin (EVANS et al., 2002; RANDALL, 2005). Patients undergoing dental procedures that cause significant bleeding require careful management of anticoagulation. It is recommended that, for procedures associated with significant bleeding, the International Normalized Ratio (INR) should be reduced to the low or subtherapeutic range and that the normal dose of oral anticoagulation should be resumed immediately after the procedure. Most dental procedures can be carried out safely with an INR of up to 4.0 without having to suspend anticoagulation, but for patients with any heart disease associated with hypertension, such as prosthetic valves, the INR can be considered at 3.5 (RANDALL, 2005; WARURTON AND CACAMESE, 2006).

In addition, the use of anti-hypertensive drugs means that these patients are closely linked to dental care, since some drugs can cause adverse effects in the oral cavity, and it is therefore extremely important to know the possible local and/or systemic complications that may arise as a result of the drug therapy used in hypertensive individuals (COSTA et al., 2013).

The administration of antihypertensive medication is described as the responsibility of the specialist doctor (ANDRADE, 2014). GEALH and FRANCO, (2006); LÚCIO and BARRETO, (2012), show that the dental surgeon can administer this class of medication in the event of a hypertensive emergency in his office, with oral captopril being recommended.

Chapter 4

4 DISCUSSION

A review of the relevant literature showed that hypertension increases cardiovascular risk and is one of the main contributors to strokes and coronary heart disease in Brazil and worldwide (GLOBAL ATLAS ON CARDIOVASCULAR DISEASES PREVENTION AND CONTROL 2011; WHO, 2010; SOCIEDADE BRASILEIRA DE HIPERTENSÁO, 2015). Access to primary care cardiovascular risk assessment and essential medications for cardiovascular risk reduction can improve the health outcomes of people with hypertension (WHO, 2010). Policies to reduce salt consumption can change the distribution of the prevalence of the population with hypertension, so that there will be a consequent reduction in cardiovascular risk (WHO, 2007). Clinical studies by the Brazilian Society of Cardiology (SBC) have shown that the detection, treatment and control of hypertension are fundamental to reducing cardiovascular events (BRAZILIAN SOCIETY OF CARDIOLOGY, 2006). In Brazil, 14 population studies carried out over the last fifteen years with 14,783 individuals (BP < 140/90 mmHg) revealed low levels of BP control (19.6%), which means that these rates are probably overestimated, mainly due to the heterogeneity of the studies carried out during this period. A comparison of the frequencies of knowledge, treatment and control, respectively, in the Brazilian studies by Rosário et al. (2009) with the frequencies obtained in 44 studies from 35 countries in the study by Pereira et al, 2009, revealed similar rates in relation to knowledge (52.3% *vs.* 59.1%), but significantly higher rates in Brazil in relation to treatment and control (34.9% and 13.7% *vs.* 67.3% and 26.1%), especially in inland municipalities with extensive FHP coverage, which demonstrates that the concentrated efforts of health professionals, scientific societies and government agencies are fundamental to achieving acceptable targets for the treatment and control of hypertension (ROSÁRIO, et al., 2009).

Figures compiled by the World Health Organization in 2010 suggest that the prevalence of non-communicable diseases and the resulting number of related deaths are expected to increase substantially in the future, particularly in low- and middle-income countries, due to population growth and ageing, together with economic transition, occupational and environmental risk factors. This is borne out by non-communicable diseases, such as SAH, which already disproportionately affect low- and middle-income countries and by current projections which indicate that, by 2020, the greatest increases in mortality from such non-communicable diseases will occur in Africa and other low- and middle-income countries (WHO, 2008).

There are many studies estimating the prevalence of SAH in the world, but few in Brazil and most of them are unreliable. Sometimes the discrepant prevalence rates in these studies can be explained by the different methodologies applied, such as the different definitions and cut-off points for defining SAH, as well as variations in the target population (different age groups, samples with selected groups), number of visits to measure blood pressure, as well as the racial, cultural and socio-economic variations of the populations in the different regions studied (NEDER, BORGES, 2006). In this context, Pereira et al. (2007) observed that the prevalence of pre-hypertension is higher in younger individuals than in the elderly (> 60 years), while the prevalence of hypertension increases with age in both sexes, but the adjusted prevalences of both pre-hypertension and hypertension were significantly higher in men than in women. It is also noteworthy that women showed greater knowledge of being hypertensive, had a higher rate of treatment and were better controlled. PASSOS et al. (2006) concluded, after analysis, that hypertension in adults in Brazil has reached levels that demonstrate the need for immediate intervention by Public Health, both in health care and in taking preventive measures aimed at a global approach to risk factors for cardiovascular diseases.

Lifestyle changes for patients with borderline BP below 140/90 mmHg are associated with a reduction in cardiovascular complications. It should be noted that for patients at medium, high and very high cardiovascular risk, regardless of BP, this non-drug intervention is also valid in association with antihypertensive drugs (WHO, 2007; BAVITZ, 2006; WHO, 2010; SOCIEDADE BRASILEIRA DE HIPERTENSÁO, 2015).

NYSDJ, (2004) emphasizes the importance of a thorough anamnesis and a good preoperative assessment of patients with cardiovascular involvement, in order to minimize the risk of complications. By carrying out this prior assessment of the need for treatment and the expected limitations, patients and dentists will benefit in terms of the outcome of the planned dental care. Little et al. also emphasize the importance of identifying antihypertensive medication and the patient's adherence to the therapeutic regime, which should be questioned during the first consultation.

The use of classification systems, such as alternative risk assessment strategies like the ASA and METs (EAGLE et al., 2002; FLEISCHER,

2004; STEINHAUER et al., 2005), can help guide the treatment of patients with SAH in dental practices. However, Bavitz (2006) points out that there are no absolute black or white numbers to cut off that contraindicate the treatment of a patient with SAH. The dentist must decide whether the benefits of proceeding with a procedure outweigh any systemic risks.

In a review of the literature, authors made it clear that it is important to respect the recommendations for a good and reliable BP measurement in the doctor's office, such as the position of the patient and the cuff when checking (MACPHEE and MASSIE, 2006). INDRIAGO (2007) adds that BP should be measured a second time 5 minutes after the first recording to confirm it. Many common medical conditions such as SAH have guidelines to help with their diagnosis and treatment. These guidelines are typically formulated by recognized experts from various disciplines related to the field. For hypertension, we have guidelines that have been established in order to categorize these BP values and guide the diagnosis of SAH. The most recent Brazilian guidelines defined a new category of 120-130/80-89 mmHg as "borderline" hypertension and defined 140-159 (systolic pressure) and 90-99 (diastolic pressure) as diagnostic for stage 1 hypertension (BRAZILIAN HYPERTENSION SOCIETY, 2010).

Dental care for this patient profile should be planned from the moment the appointment is made. Short, morning appointments have been described as being well tolerated in order to reduce the chances of endogenous release of ketacolamines during the appointment, which would lead to a consequent rise in BP (LITTLE, et al., 2008). On seeing the patient in the office, the first task for the dental surgeon is to identify patients with hypertension, both diagnosed and undiagnosed. Sometimes, patients may not report a diagnosis of hypertension, however, they may report using certain herbal medicines, which are generally used to treat high BP. According to Little et al. (2008), this report may be the only way for the dentist to find out information that reveals the patient's hypertension. This justifies the importance of prior knowledge of antihypertensive drugs and their adverse effects (COSTA et al., 2013).

In addition to taking an anamnesis, all patients should have their blood pressure taken. Patients who are being treated for hypertension but have blood pressure above normal are more often non-cooperators, and those who are inadequately treated should be encouraged to return to their doctor. Notably, patients who have not been diagnosed with hypertension but have abnormally high blood pressure should also be encouraged by the dental surgeon to see a doctor (LITTLE et al., 2008). In the latter case, it is worth emphasizing that the dentist should not make a diagnosis of hypertension, but instead should tell the patient that their BP measurement is high, and that a doctor should assess the condition suggestive of SAH.

ANDRADE (2014) states that patients with stage 1 and stage 2 SAH should not receive dental treatment but should be referred to a doctor immediately. LITTLE et al. (2008) argue that dental treatment should only be postponed for patients with a BP above 180 over 110. LITTLE et al. (2008) base their opinion on the guidelines of the American College of Cardiology and the American Heart Association, which assess the risk of a serious event occurring in a patient with cardiovascular disease undergoing non-cardiac surgery and can be applied to non-surgical dental treatment. Despite the numerous precautions that need to be taken when receiving a patient with hypertension in the office, Little et al. (2008) add that the risk of providing routine dental treatment for most patients with high BP is very low, since in summary patients with BP <180/110 can undergo the necessary emergency dental treatment if all the preoperative and postoperative precautions are taken, both surgical and non-surgical, with a very small risk of an adverse outcome. For patients with uncontrolled BP (>180/110), elective dental treatment should be postponed so that the patient can consult a doctor and, finally, in cases of uncontrolled hypertension associated with symptoms such as chest pain, more urgent medical attention may be required. In the latter case of uncontrolled or severe hypertension, emergency dental treatment (pain, infection or bleeding) may be necessary. The NATIONAL HEART LUNG AND BLOOD INSTITUTE (2004) stresses that cases in which BP > 180/ 120 can be classified as an urgency or emergency and the patient should be referred for medical attention.

There are reports by other authors who have published and support a BP of 180/110 mmHg as the absolute cut-off for any dental treatment (AUBERTIN, 2004; RILEY AND TEREZHALMY, 2001), but they point out that this value may, in fact, be too high for patients who have had organ damage related to a previous hypertensive crisis, such as myocardial infarctions, strokes or labile angina, suggesting a medical reassessment of these cases.

For patients with no previous history of hypertension who present themselves at dental practices with a toothache, swelling and a BP in the 190/110 range, Bavitz (2006) reports that these patients are sick, anxious, desperate, and in need of emergency treatment that outweighs the presence of their high BP. It has been described that dental care can cause blood pressure to rise due to fear and anxiety related to the procedures that are carried out during dental treatment (BAVITZ, 2006). In the treatment of fearful and highly anxious patients, iatrosedation is the first alternative and pharmacosedation the second. Fear should be reduced to the lowest possible level with iatrosedation, if this level is not low enough to allow the patient to cope with the dental experience, pharmacosedation is used in addition (FRIEDMAN, 1967). Anxiolytics and sedatives can be prescribed for patients taking antihypertensive drugs, but Little et al. (2008) point out that there is a need to reduce their usual dosage. In most cases, however, iatrosedation alone can reduce fear to a functional level (FRIEDMAN, 1967).

Adverse effects of antihypertensive drugs are well described in the literature, with gingival hyperplasia standing out (BAVITZ, 2006; HERMAN et al., 2004; LITTLE et al., 2008). However, in addition to hyperplasia, the dental surgeon should be aware of pharmacological treatment with antihypertensive drugs which can also lead to xerostomia, reduced tongue mobility, difficulty in chewing and swallowing food, altered sense of taste, increased incidence of candida infections, increased caries and periodontal disease, nocturnal oral discomfort and burning sensation (CORRÊA et al., 2005).

In order to avoid complications such as bleeding in patients with SAH who use anticoagulants, there are reports in the literature of warfarin or any other drug being suspended for oral surgery (EVANS et al., 2002; RANDALL, 2005). However, the current trend is to request follow-up tests from the doctor in charge, such as a coagulogram. The risk of lowering the INR value compared to the risk of thromboembolic events should be assessed in patients with cardiovascular impairment, especially mitral valve patients, and a possible change/reduction in the dose of the patient's medication should only be requested if it is really necessary for successful surgery (RANDALL, 2005; WARURTON AND CACAMESE, 2006). A rational approach in such patients, especially if BP is high, is to perform one or two extractions and check for good coagulation before continuing (WARURTON AND CACAMESE, 2006).

Although the interaction between antihypertensive drugs and general anesthetic agents is primarily the responsibility of the anesthesiologist, dentists should be aware of intra- and post-operative control. When control of hypertension becomes a challenge in hypertensive patients who require emergency care, clinical treatment in an outpatient setting is limited, dental treatment under general anesthesia should be considered (GLICK, 2004).

Malamed (2013) reports, however, that many doctors are unfamiliar with the doses of epinephrine used by dentists, and often inappropriately advise them to proceed with treatment and not use adrenaline. The author goes on to say that the primary responsibility for patient care rests solely in the hands of the person carrying out the treatment, and not the one giving the advice. Costa el al. concluded that the very act of anesthetizing causes enough apprehension to stimulate variations in blood pressure, further increasing the patient's blood pressure, regardless of the type of local anesthetic used, with or without a vasoconstrictor. It should be noted that although there are several studies on the effects of anesthetics on patients with SAH during dental treatment, they are contradictory as to safe doses of anesthetics that would have minimal effect on coronary circulation, blood pressure and heart rate (CASTRO, et al, 1980; SUNADA et al., 1996). Except perhaps the ASA Class IV patient with MET capacity 4, or a person who has recently used cocaine, there is no absolute contraindication to the use of adrenaline in the 0.04 to 0.06 mg range. Rarely does a dentist have to give more than two tubes of local anesthesia with epinephrine at the same time (BAVITZ, 2006). It should be noted that if several quadrants are planned for dental treatment, it is necessary to check vital signs after one quadrant has been completed in order to assess the possibility of safely proceeding to the next.

Attention should also be paid when prescribing drugs by dentists due to the possible interaction of these drugs with the antihypertensive agents the patient is already taking. Care should be taken in the case of NSAIDs, which are more preferred in dentists' routine prescriptions, as they reduce the action of most antihypertensive drugs (BAVITZ, 2006). This effect of compromising the efficacy of antihypertensive drugs is mainly due to the prolonged use of NSAIDs, which should be considered if these drugs are used for analgesia, although the use of NSAIDs for a few days does not have much influence in practice (LITTLE et al., 2008).

BAVITZ (2006) adds that the dentist should document BP values and then refer patients with high BP numbers for immediate medical attention after all emergency dental care has been provided, and emphasizes that the dentist should be encouraged to check with current references when questions arise about medications, their adverse effects and drug-to-drug interactions. Lúcio and Barreto (2012) add the possibility of dentists administering the antihypertensive Captopril when faced with a hypertensive crisis in the office. In view of all the literature reports presented and the characteristics of the current population, the dental surgeon must be trained to identify SAH and its comorbidities, plan treatment, carry out treatment and deal with possible hypertensive crisis situations with the confidence of prior scientific knowledge, creating an evidence-based care protocol.

CONCLUSION

- High BP is the result of inflexible narrow arteries, a high heart rate, increased blood volume, stronger heart contractions, or any combination of the above.
- SAH is one of the most important risk factors for the development of various cardiovascular and cerebrovascular diseases and for kidney failure, and is the leading cause of death globally today.
- Guidelines are well-established and frequently updated about SAH and serve to guide the professionals who receive these patients in their practices to assess the risk of a serious event occurring.
- The dental surgeon, as a health professional, plays an extremely important role in diagnosing systemic diseases such as hypertension.
- The dental surgeon should apply measures to reduce the anxiety associated with dental treatment as much as possible for all patients, especially those with SAH, through pharmacological or non-pharmacological strategies.
- Dental surgeons should be aware that they may see patients with hypertension in their work environment who may experience adverse effects from antihypertensive drugs, who need prescriptions for drugs that may interact with antihypertensive drugs and who are potentially prone to developing medical emergencies, such as a hypertensive crisis.
- Identify, diagnose, plan and provide care for hypertensive patients with scientific basis, should be a skill of today's dental surgeon.

REFERENCES

ANDRADE E.D. Terapéutica Medicamentosa em Odontología. 3a Ed. Sao Paulo: Editora Artes Médicas Ltda. p.35-45, 2014.

ARSATI F.; MONTALLI V.A.; FLÓRIO F.M.; RAMACCIATO J.C.; DA CUNHA F.L.; CECANHO R. et al. Brazilian dentists' attitudes about medical emergencies during Dental treatment. **Int Dent Educ**. v.74; n.6, p.661-666, 2010.

AUBERTIN M.A. The hypertensive patient in dental practice: updated recommendations for classification, prevention, monitoring, and dental management. **Gen Dent.** v.52, n.6, p.544-52. 2004

BARCLAY L.; VEGA C. Updated guidelines address use of oral appliances for sleep apnea. **Sleep.** V.29. p. 240-3, 2006.

BRAND HS. Cardiovascular responses in patients and dentists during dental treatment. **International Dental Journal.** v.49, n.1, p.60-66, 1999.

CARNEVALLI ARAÚJO AND ARAGÂO ARAÚJO. Etiopathogenesis of arterial hypertension, risks and preventive measures to be employed in dental care for hypertensive patients. Belém- Pará, p 4-25, 2001.

CASTRO A.L; CARVALHO A.C.P; FONSECA L.G.N. Local anesthetics: types, mechanisms of action, absorption and accidents. Rev Cient. Ass. Prudent Ens. Cult.; 1, 2: 63-77, 1980.

CESARINO C.B.; CIPULLO J.P; MARTIN J.F.V.; CIORLIA L.A.; GODOY M.R.P; CORDEIRO J.A.; RODRIGUES I.C. Prevalence and sociodemographic factors in hypertensive patients in Sao José do Rio Preto. **Arq Bras Card**. v.91, n.1, p.31-35, 2008.

CORRÊA T. et al. Systemic arterial hypertension: updates on its epidemiology, diagnosis and treatment. **Arq Med ABC**. 2005; 31(2):91-101.

COSTA A. et al. Dental conduct in hypertensive patients. **Revista Brasileira de Ciencias da Saúde.** v. 17, n.3, p. 287-292, 2013.

CONROTTO D; CARBONE M; CARROZZO M; et al. Ciclosporin vs. clobetasol in the topical man- agement of atrophic and erosive oral lichen planus: a double-blind, randomized controlled trial. **Br J Dermatol.** V.154, n.1, p.139-45, 2006.

CHOBANIAN A.V; BAKRIS G.L; BLACK H.R; CUSHMAN W.C; GREEN L.A; IZZO J.R. J.L. et al. The Seventh Report of the Joint National Committee on Prevention, Detection, Evaluation, and Treatment of High Blood Pressure: the JNC 7 report. **JAMA**. 289:2560-72, 2003.

DANAEI G. et al. National, regional, and global trends in systolic blood pressure since 1980: Systematic analysis of health examination surveys and epidemiological studies with 786 country-years and 54 million participants. ***Lancet***. v.377, n.9765, p.568-577, 2011.

DE GREEFF A; LORD I; WILTON A; SEED P; COLEMAN A.J; SHENNAN AH. Calibration accuracy of hospital-based non-invasive blood pressure measuring devices. **J Hum Hypertens. V.**24, n.1, p. 58-63, 2010.

Department of Surgical Specialties. University of Nebraska Medical Center, College of Dentistry. **Dent Clin N Am**. v.50, p. 547-562, 2006
IV BRAZILIAN GUIDELINES ON ARTERIAL HYPERTENSION. **Arq.Bras. Cardiolog**. 82, suppl. IV: 1-14, 2004.
EAGLE K.A; BERGER P.B; CALKINS H; et al. ACC/AHA guideline update for perioperative car- diovascular evaluation for noncardiac surgerydexecutive summary. A report to the American College of Cardiology/American Heart Association Task Force on practice guidelines. **J Am Coll Cardiol.** V.39, n.3, p.543-51, 2002.
Epidemiology and Health Services. Hypertension in Brazil: prevalence estimates from population-based studies. **Estimativa de Prevalência de Hipertensao no Brasil.** v. 15. n.1 - jan/mar, 2006.
EVANS I.L.; SAYERS M.S.; GIBBONS A.J; et al. Can warfarin be continued during dental extrac- tion? Results of a randomized controlled trial. Br J Oral Maxillofac Surg. v.40, n.3, p.248-52, 2002.
FLEISCHER L.A. Preoperative evaluation of the patient with hypertension. JAMA. v. 287 p. 2043-6, 2002.
Friedman, N. Iatrosedation. ***"Emergencies in Dental Practice", 1967.***
FRIEDMAN N.; WOOD G.J. An evaluation of the iatrosedative process for treating dental fear. **Compend Contin Educ Dent**. v.19, n.4, p.434-442, 1998.
FUCHS F.D. Systemic arterial hypertension. In: Duncan BB, Schmidt MI, Giugliani ERJ, et al. Outpatient medicine: evidence-based primary care guidelines. Porto Alegre: Artmed; 2004. p.641-56.
GEALH W.C.; FRANCO W.P.G. Atendimento odontológico ao paciente hipertenso protocolo baseado no VII JCN. **J Bras Clin Odontol Int-** Special edition, 2006.
Global health risks: mortality and burden of disease attributable to selected major risks. Geneva, **World Health Organization**, 2009.
GLICK M. The new blood pressure guidelines: a digest. **J Am Dent Assoc.** v.135, p.585-6, 2004.
GROSSMAN E.; NADLER M.; SHARABI Y.; et al. Antianxiety treatment in patients with excessive hypertension. **Am J Hypertens.** v.18,1, p.174-7, 2005.
GUS M. Clinical trials in isolated systolic hypertension. **Rev Bras Hipertens.** v.16, n.1, p.26-28, 2009.
HERMAN W.W; KONZELMAN J.L; PRISANT L.M. New national guideline son hypertension: a summary for dentistry. **J Am Dent Assoc.** v.135, p.576-84, 2004.
KAPLAN N. Systemic hypertension: Mechanisms and Diagnosis. In Zipes D, Libby P, Bonow R, Braunwald E (eds). Braunwald's Hart Desease: A Textbook of Cardiolovascular Medicine, 7 th ed. Philadelphia, Elsevier, 2005.
KLEIN C.H; SILVA N.A; NOGUEIRA A.R; BLOCH K.V; CAMPOS L.H. Arterial hypertension in Ilha do Governador, Rio de Janeiro, Brazil: I.

Methodology. Cadernos de Saúde Pública. v.II, n. 3, p.389-394, 1995.
KNOLL-KOHLER E.; FRIE A.; BECKER J.; et al. Changes in plasma epinephrine concentration after dental infiltration anesthesia with different doses of epinephrine. **J Dent Res**. v.68, p.1098-101, 1989.
INDRIAGO A. Dental management of hypertensive patients. **Acta Odontológica Venezolana**. Caracas, Venezuela. V. 45 N. 1, 2007.
JARDIM P.C.V; PEIXOTO M.R; MONEGO E; MOREIRA H; VITORINO P.V.O; SOUZA W.S.B.S; SCALA L.C.N. Hipertensâo arterial e alguns fatores de risco em uma capital brasileira. **Arq Bras Card**. v.88 n.4, p.452457, 2007.
LITTLE J.; FALACE D.; MILLER C.; RHODUS N. Dental management of the clinically compromised patient. 7th Edition. Rio de Janeiro: Editora Elsevier, p 37-50, 2008.
LÚCIO C.S.P., BARRETO C.R., Medical emergencies in the dental office and the insecurity of professionals. Brazilian Journal of Health Sciences. Vol 16. NO 2 P 267-272, 2012.
MALAMED F.; Manual of local anesthesia - pharmacology of local anesthetics and pharmacology of vasoconstrictors. 6th Ed. Rio de Janeiro: Editora Elsevier, p27-54, 2013.
MANCIA G.; SEGA R.; BRAVI C.; DE VITO G.; VALAGUSSA F.; CESANA G. et al. Ambulatory blood pressure normality: results from the PAMELA study. **J Hypertens**. V.13(12 Pt 1), p.1377-1390, Dec, 1995.
MANCIA G.; FACCHETTI R.; BOMBELLI M.; GRASSI G., SEGA R. Long-term risk of mortality associated with selective and combined elevation in office, home, and ambulatory blood pressure. Hypertension. v.47, n.5, p.846-853, 2006.
MANCIA G.; DE BACKER G.; DOMINICZAK A. et al. ESH-ESC Task Force on the Management of Arterial Hypertension. 2007 ESH-ESC Practice Guidelines for the Management of Arterial Hypertension: ESH-ESC Task Force on the Management of Arterial Hypertension. **J Hypertens**. v.25, n.9, p.1751-1762, 2007.
MENIN C. et al. Evaluation of hypertensive patients in the surgery clinic of the third year of the dentistry course at Cesumar. v. 08, n.2, p. 147-156, Jul./Dec. 2006.
MCPHEE SJ, MASSIE BM. HYPERTENSION. IN: TIERNEY LM, MCPHEE SJ, PAPADAKIS MA, et al, editors. **Current medical diagnosis & treatment**. New York: mcgraw-hill, 2006.
MISHIMA R.; KUDO T.; TSUNETSUGU Y; et al. Effects of sounds generated by a dental turbine and a stream on regional cerebral blood flow and cardiovascular responses. **Odontology**. V.92, p.54-60, 2004.
NATIONAL HEART LUNG AND BLOOD INSTITUTE. Morbidity and Mortality Chartbook and Cardiovascular, Lung, and Blood Diseases. Bethesda, Md, NHLBI, 2004).
OLIVEIRA A., SIMONE J., RIBEIRO R. Hypertensive patients and anesthesia in dentistry: should we use local anesthetics associated or not

with vasoconstrictors? **HU Magazine**. Juiz de Fora, v.36, n.1, p. 69- 75, jan./mar.2010.
WORLD HEALTH ORGANIZATION. **Innovative care for chronic conditions**: structural components **for** action: world report. Brasilia, 2003.
LIFSHE F. M. Evaluation of and Treatment Considerations for the Dental Patient with Cardiac Disease. **NYSDJ.** p. 16-19. November, 2004.
LÜDERS S, SCHRADER J, BERGER J ET AL. PHARAO STUDY GROUP. The PHARAO study: prevention of hypertension with the angiotensin-converting enzyme inhibitor ramipril in patients with highnormal blood pressure: a prospective, randomized, controlled prevention trial of the German Hypertension League. **J Hypertens**. v.26, n.7, p.14871496, Jul, 2008.
PARATI, G.; STERGIOU G.S.; ASMAR R., et al. European Society of Hypertension guidelines for blood pressure monitoring at home: a summary report of the Second International Consensus Conference on Home Blood Pressure Monitoring. **J Hypertens**, v.26, p.1505-1526, 2008.
PASSOS, V.M.A.; ASSIS T.D.; BARRETO S.M. Hipertensao arterial no Brasil: estimativa de prevalência a partir de estudos de base populacional. **Epidemiologia e Serviços de Saúde**. v. 15, n.1, p.35 - 45, 2006.
PEET M. The treatment of anxiety with beta-blocking drugs. **Postgrad Med J**. v. 64, Suppl 2, p.45-49, 1988.
PEREIRA, M; LUNET, N; AZEVEDO, A; BARROS, H. Differences in prevalence, awareness, treatment and control of hypertension between developing and developed countries. **J Hypertension**. v.27, n.5, p.963-975, 2009.
RANDALL C. Surgical management of the primary care dental patient on warfarin. **Dent Up-date**. V.32; n.7, p.414-6, 419-20, 423-4, 2005.
REDDY, K.S; YUSUF, S. Emerging epidemic of cardiovascular diseases in developing countries. Circulation. V.97, p.596-601, 1998.
RIDKER P.M.; LIBBY P. Risk factors for atherothombotic disease In Zipes D, Libby P, Bonow R, Braunwald E (eds). Braunwald**'s Heart Disease,** Philadelphia, Elsevier, 2005.
ROSÁRIO, T.M; SCALA, L.C.N.S; FRANÇA, G.V.A; PEREIRA, M.R.G; Jardim P.C.B.V. Prevalence, control and treatment of systemic arterial hypertension in Nobres, MT. **Arq Bras Card**. V.93, n.6, p.672-678, 2009.
RILEY C.K.; TEREZHALMY G.T. The patient with hypertension. Quintessence. V.32, p.671-90, 2001.
SANTELLO J.L.; AMODEO C. Application and usefulness of ABPM in large hypertension studies. In: Mion JD, Oigman W, Nobre Fernando. ABPM - Ambulatory Blood Pressure Monitoring. Sao Paulo: Editora Atheneu; 3rd edition. p.141-147, 2004.
SCHAIRA V. R. L. Evaluation of cardiovascular parameters in hypertensive patients undergoing dental treatment under vasoconstrictor anesthesia. Piracibaba, 2005.
SILVESTRE F.J.; SALVADOR-MARTÍNEZ I.; BAUTISTA D.;

SILVESTRE-RANGIL J. Clinical study of hemodynamic changes during extraction in controlled hypertensive patients. **Med Oral Patol Oral Cir Bucal**, v.16, n.3, p.354-358, 2011.
BRAZILIAN SOCIETY OF HYPERTENSION; BRAZILIAN SOCIETY OF CARDIOLOGY; BRAZILIAN SOCIETY OF NEPHROLOGY. IV Brazilian Guidelines on Hypertension. Arq Bras Cardiol. V.82(Supl 4), p. 7-22, 2004.
BRAZILIAN SOCIETY OF CARDIOLOGY. V Brazilian Hypertension Guidelines. **Arq Bras Cardiol.** Feb: 1-48, 2006.
BRAZILIAN SOCIETY OF CARDIOLOGY / BRAZILIAN SOCIETY OF HYPERTENSION / BRAZILIAN SOCIETY OF NEPHROLOGY. VI Brazilian Hypertension Guidelines. Arq Bras Cardiol 2010; 95(1 supl.1): 1-51
STEINHAUER T.; BSOUL S.A.; TEREZHALMY G.T. Risk stratification and dental management of the patient with cardiovascular diseases. Part II: oral disease burden and principles of dental management. **Quintessence Int.** v.36, n.3, p.209-27, 2005.
SJOSTROM C.; LINDBERG E;. ELMASRY A;. HAGG A.; SVARDSUDD K.; JANSON C. Prevalence of sleep apnoea and snoring in hypertensive men: a population based study. **Thorax**. v.57, n.7, p.602-607, 2002.
SUNADA K, NAKAMURA K, YAMASHIRO M. Clinically safe dosage of felypressin for patients with essential hypertension. **Anesth Prog.** V.43, p.108-115,1996.
WARBURTON, G.; CACCAMESE, J.F. VALVULAR HEART DISEASE AND HEART FAILURE. **Dent Clin N Am.** v.50, n.4 P.93-512, 2006.
World Health Organization. The global burden of disease: 2004 update. Geneva, 2008.
World Health Organization. *Prevention of cardiovascular disease: Guidelines for assessment and management of car- diovascular risk.* Geneva, WHO, 2007.
World Health Organization. *Global health risks: Mortality and burden of disease attributable to selected major risks*. Geneva, WHO, 2009.
World Health Organization. *Global status report on non-communicable diseases 2010*. Geneva, WHO, 2010.
WILLIAMS SA, MICHELSON EL, CAIN VA, YANG M, NESBITT SD, EGAN BM et al; TROPHY Study Investigators. An evaluation of the effects of an angiotensin receptor blocker on health-related quality of life in patients with high-normal blood pressure (prehypertension) in the Trial of Preventing Hypertension (TROPHY). **J Clin Hypertens.** v.10, n.6, p.436-442, Jun, 2008.
Williams B. The year in hypertension. **JACC**. v.55, n.1, p.66-73, 2010.

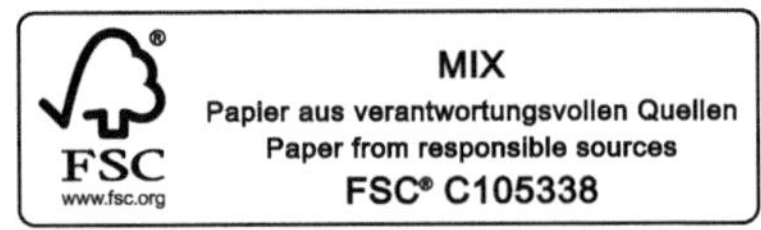

Printed by Books on Demand GmbH, Norderstedt / Germany